Marvin the DINOSAUR
Who wouldn't go to School

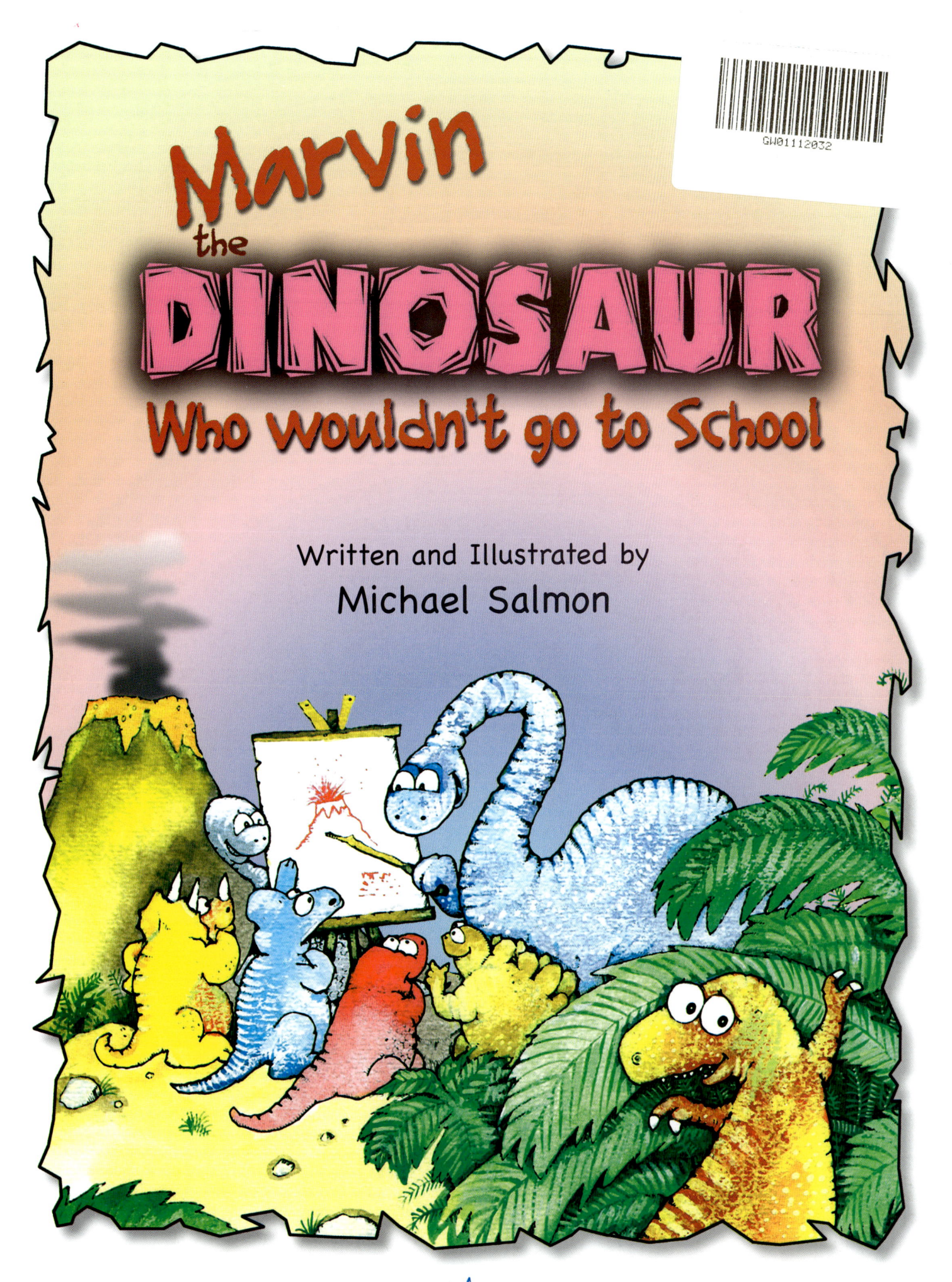

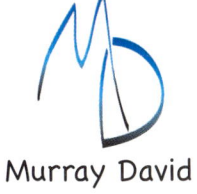

Written and Illustrated by
Michael Salmon

Murray David

How to pronounce the dinosaur name in this book

Tyrannosaurus Rex (Tyrant Lizard King)
TIE-RAN-UH-SAW-RUS REX

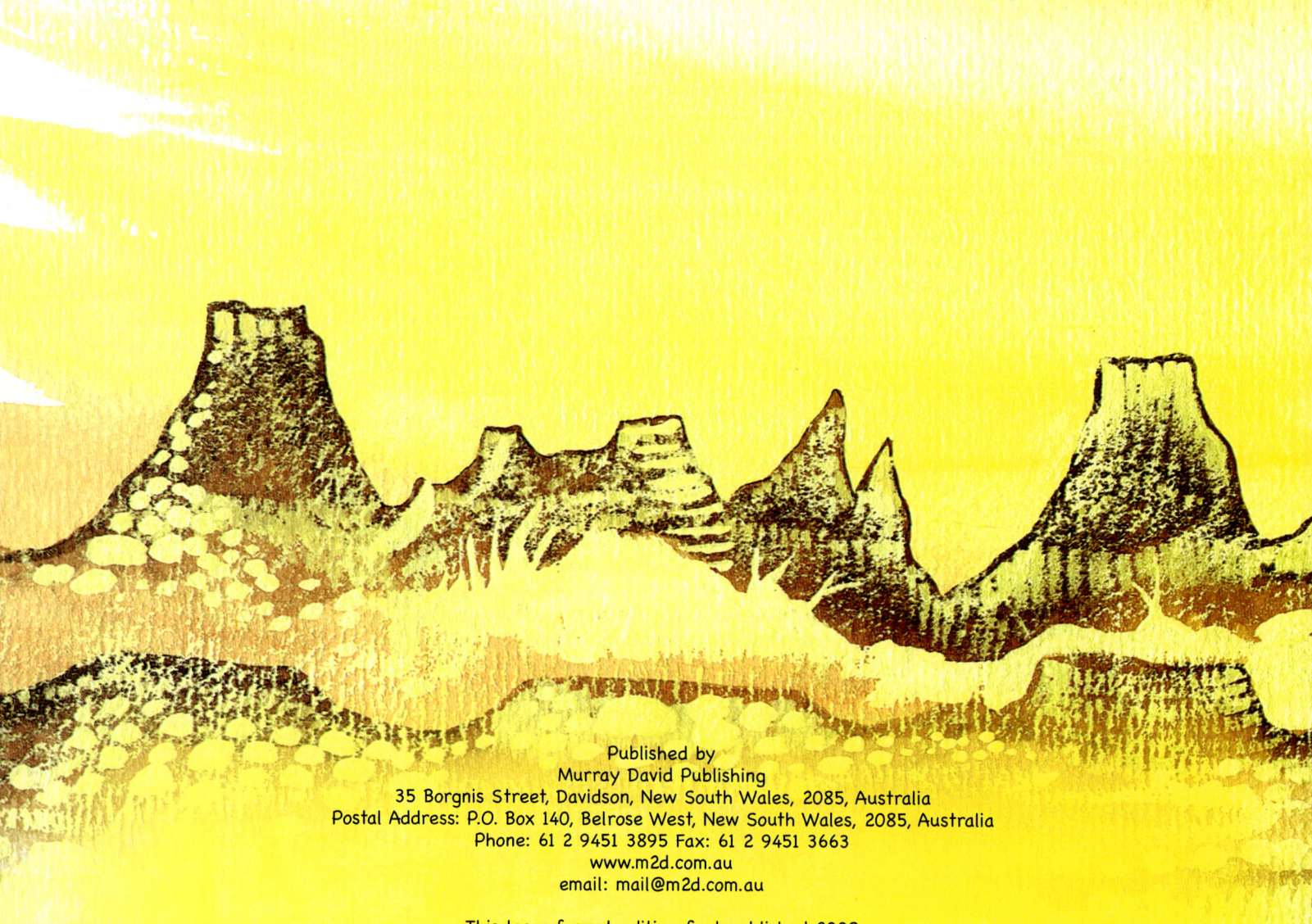

Published by
Murray David Publishing
35 Borgnis Street, Davidson, New South Wales, 2085, Australia
Postal Address: P.O. Box 140, Belrose West, New South Wales, 2085, Australia
Phone: 61 2 9451 3895 Fax: 61 2 9451 3663
www.m2d.com.au
email: mail@m2d.com.au

This large format edition first published 2008
Publishing Director: Marion Child
Marketing Director: David Jenkins
Executive Director: David Forsythe
Designed by Emma Sutton
Digital photography by the late James Young
Copyright © Monster Promotions Pty Ltd, 2008
Copyright © in layout M2D Publishing Pty Ltd, 2008
ISBN: 978-1-876411-52-7

Printed in Indonesia

All rights reserved. No part of this publication may be reproduced, stored in a retrieval system, or transmitted in any form or by any means, electronic, photocopying, recording or otherwise without prior permission in writing from Murray David Publishing.

Tyrannosaurus Rex

The tyrannosaurus rex is probably the best-known dinosaur of all time. It was the biggest, fiercest, most powerful meat-eating land animal that ever lived.

It could weigh as much as a large elephant and when it stood up it was about 6m (20ft) tall (higher than a big semi-trailer!).

Tyrannosaurus rex had a massive head with a mouth full of long curved teeth—just like knife blades. It had a large body and strong legs with enormous claws on its toes. However, its arms were very short and each hand had only two fingers. It is thought that the arms may have stopped their bodies from sliding forward as they stood up after resting.

The other dinosaurs would usually do their very best to stay out of the way of this hunter.

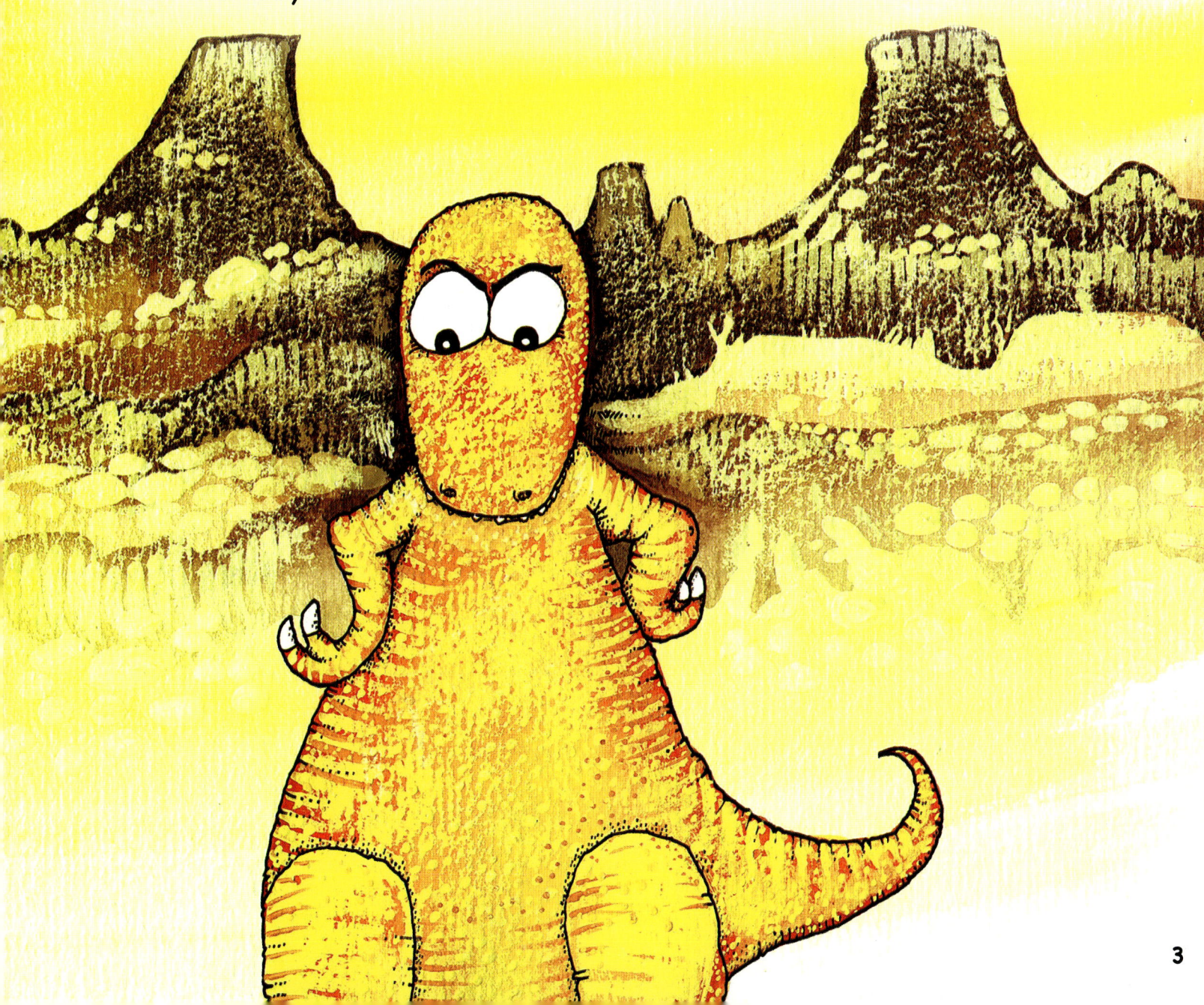

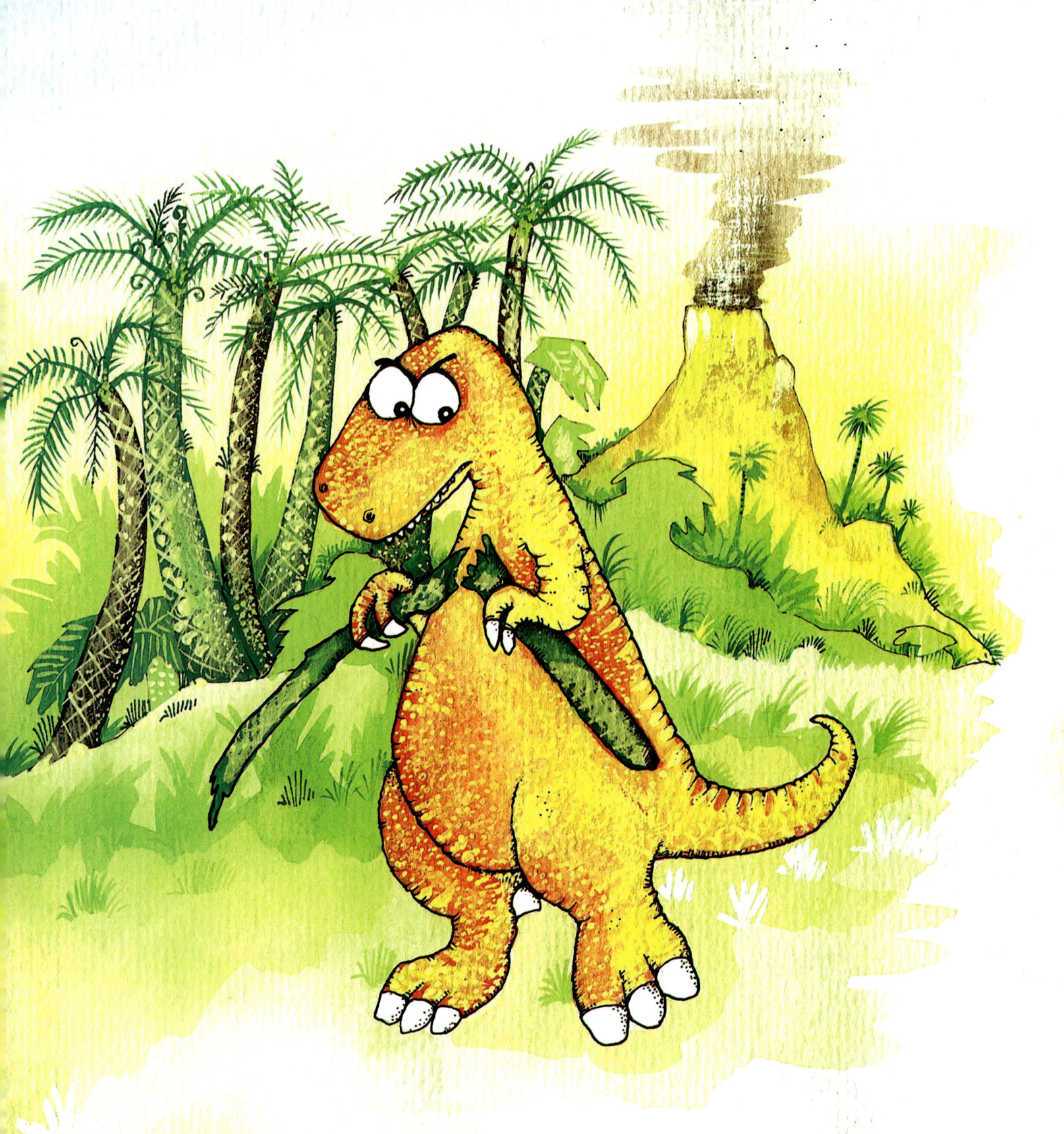

MARVIN was a young tyrannosaurus rex with a problem...he had a bad temper.

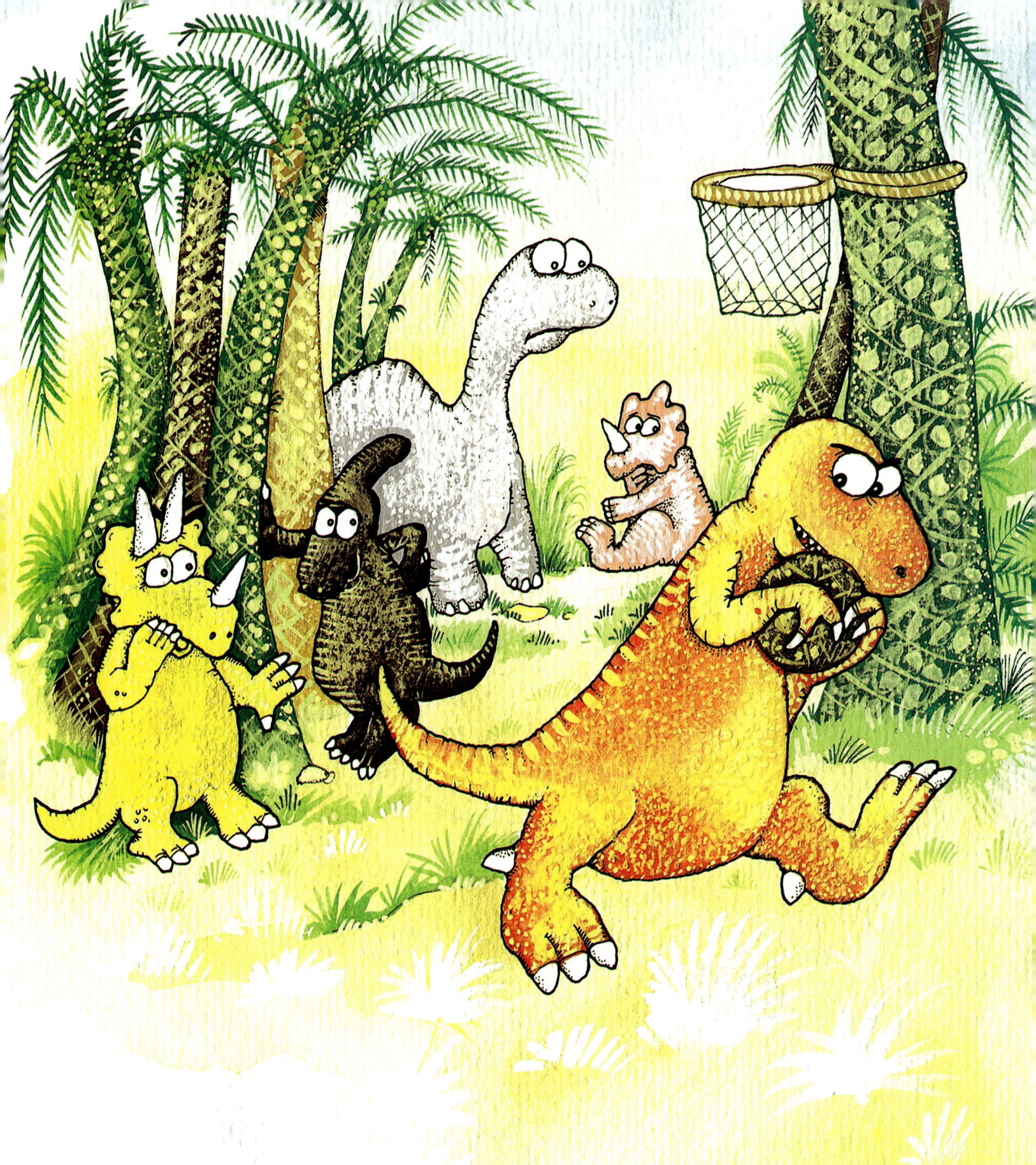

When Marvin played basketball and he missed the net, he would pick up the ball and run away with it!

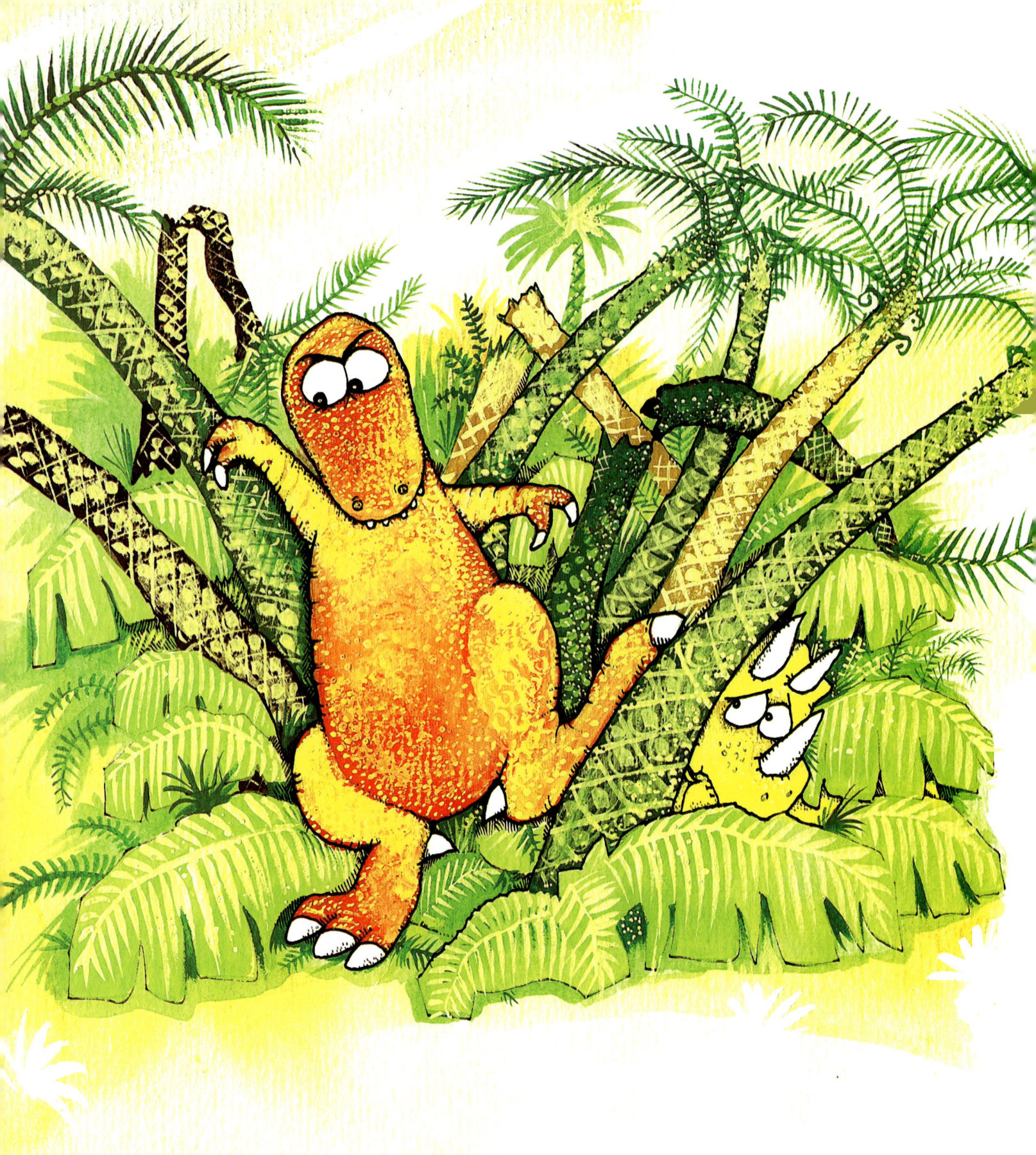

When Marvin played hide-and-seek in the forest, the other dinosaurs would let him see where they were hiding, because if Marvin couldn't find them, he would knock the trees down!

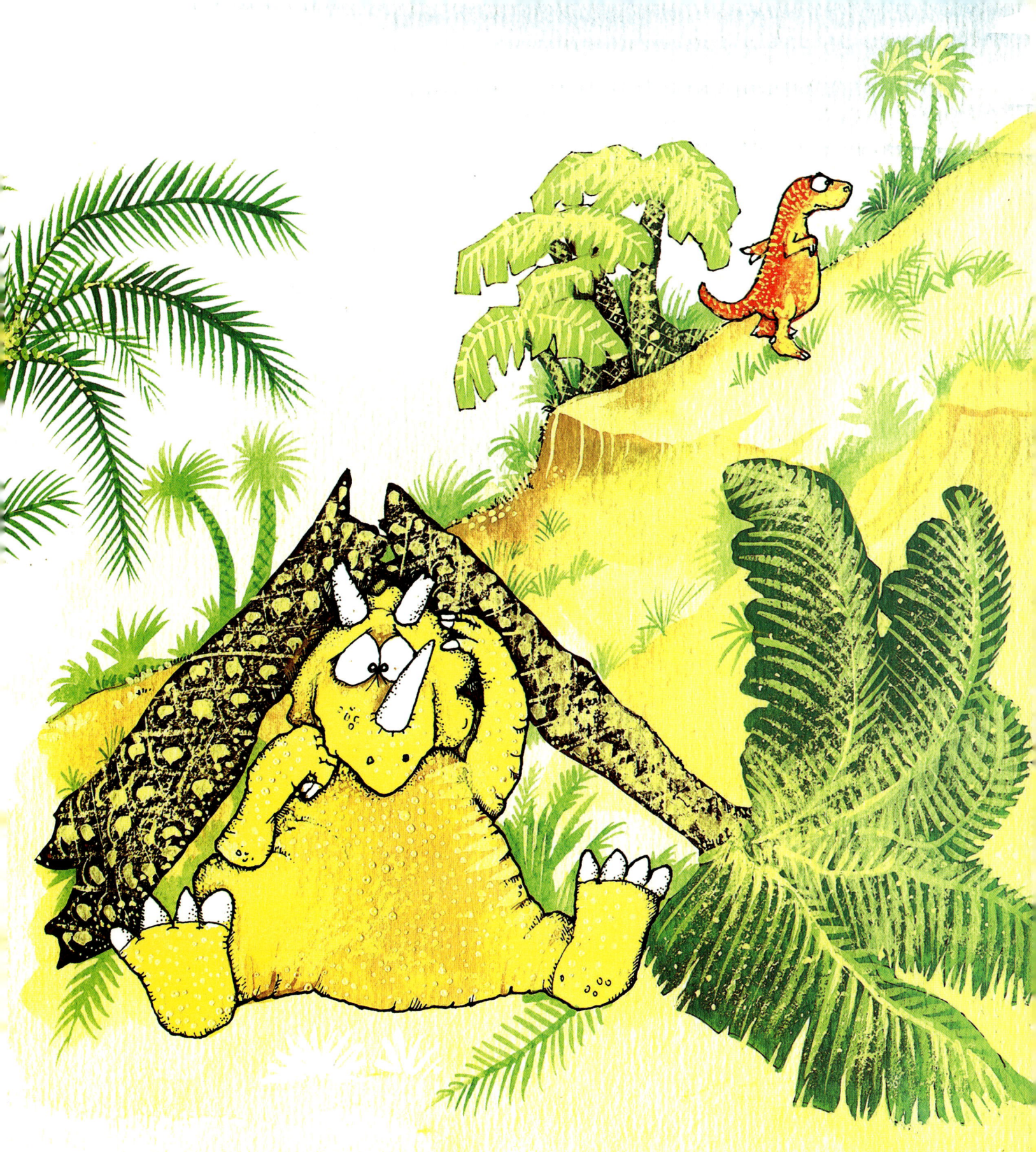

It was best to play games when Marvin was **NOT** around.

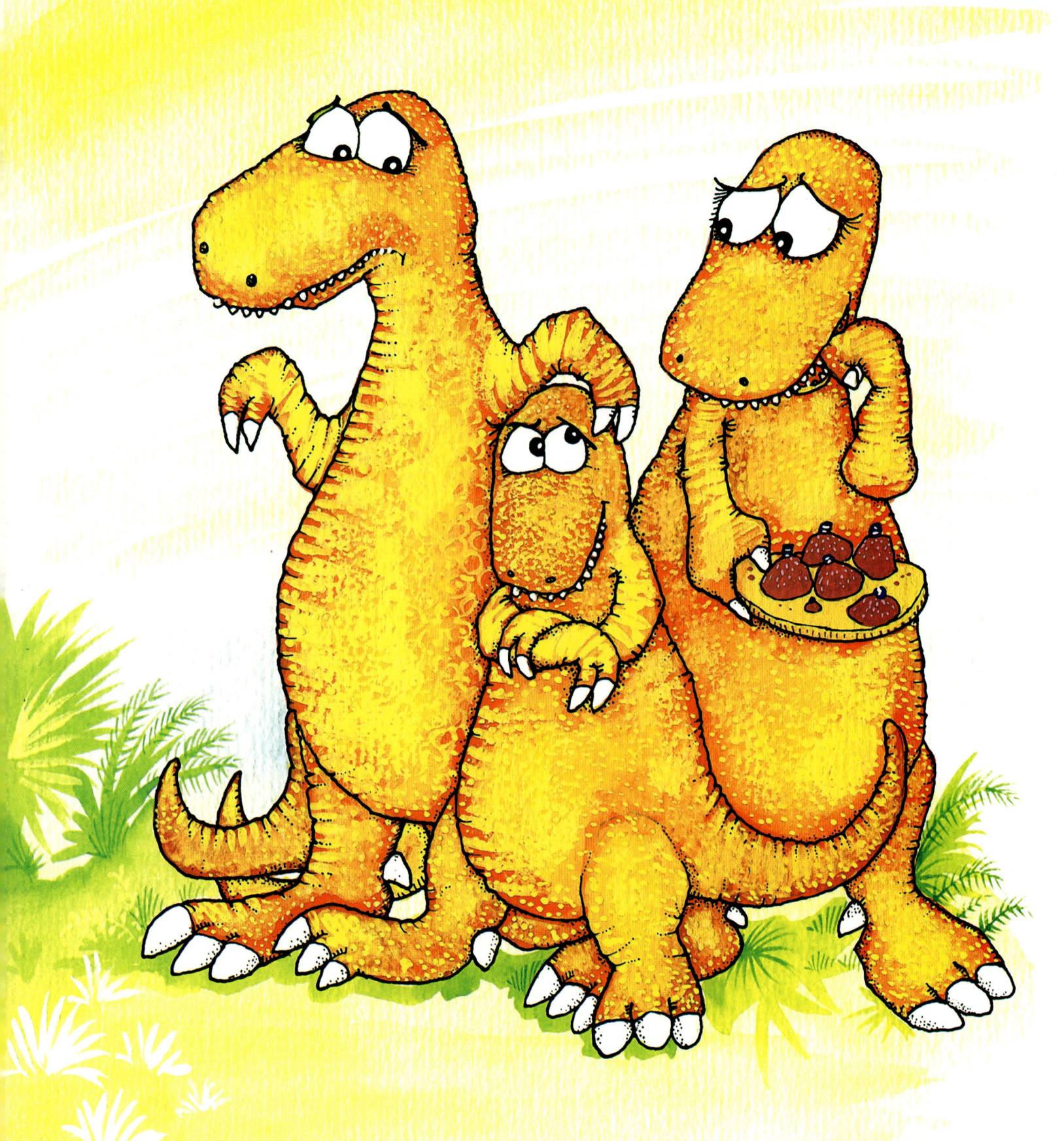

Marvin's parents were very worried about their son's bad temper...after all, Marvin always got everything he wanted!

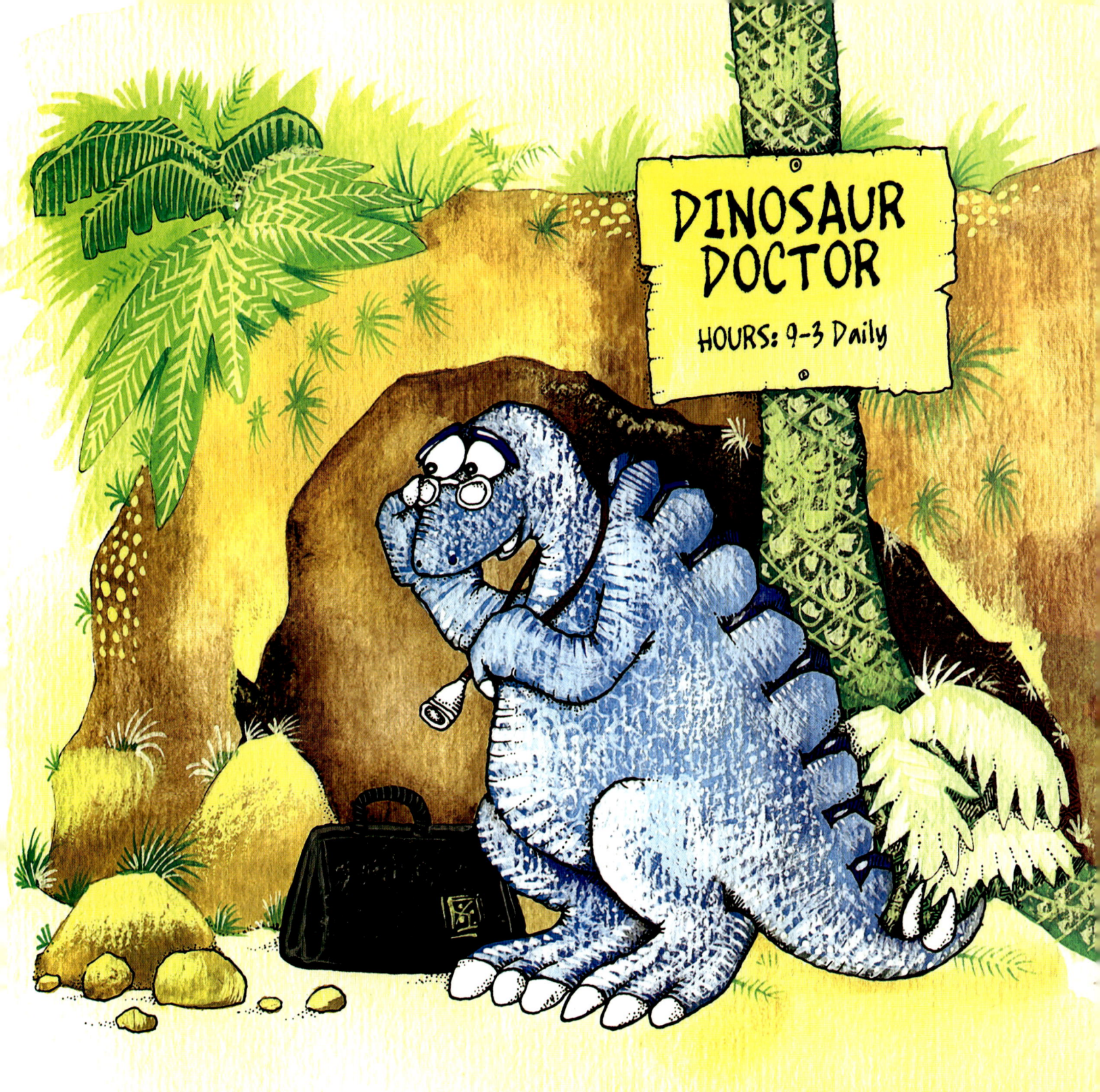

They took him to the old dinosaur doctor. 'There's nothing wrong with your son', said the old doctor. 'He just needs more to do. Your son is old enough for school and school starts tomorrow!'

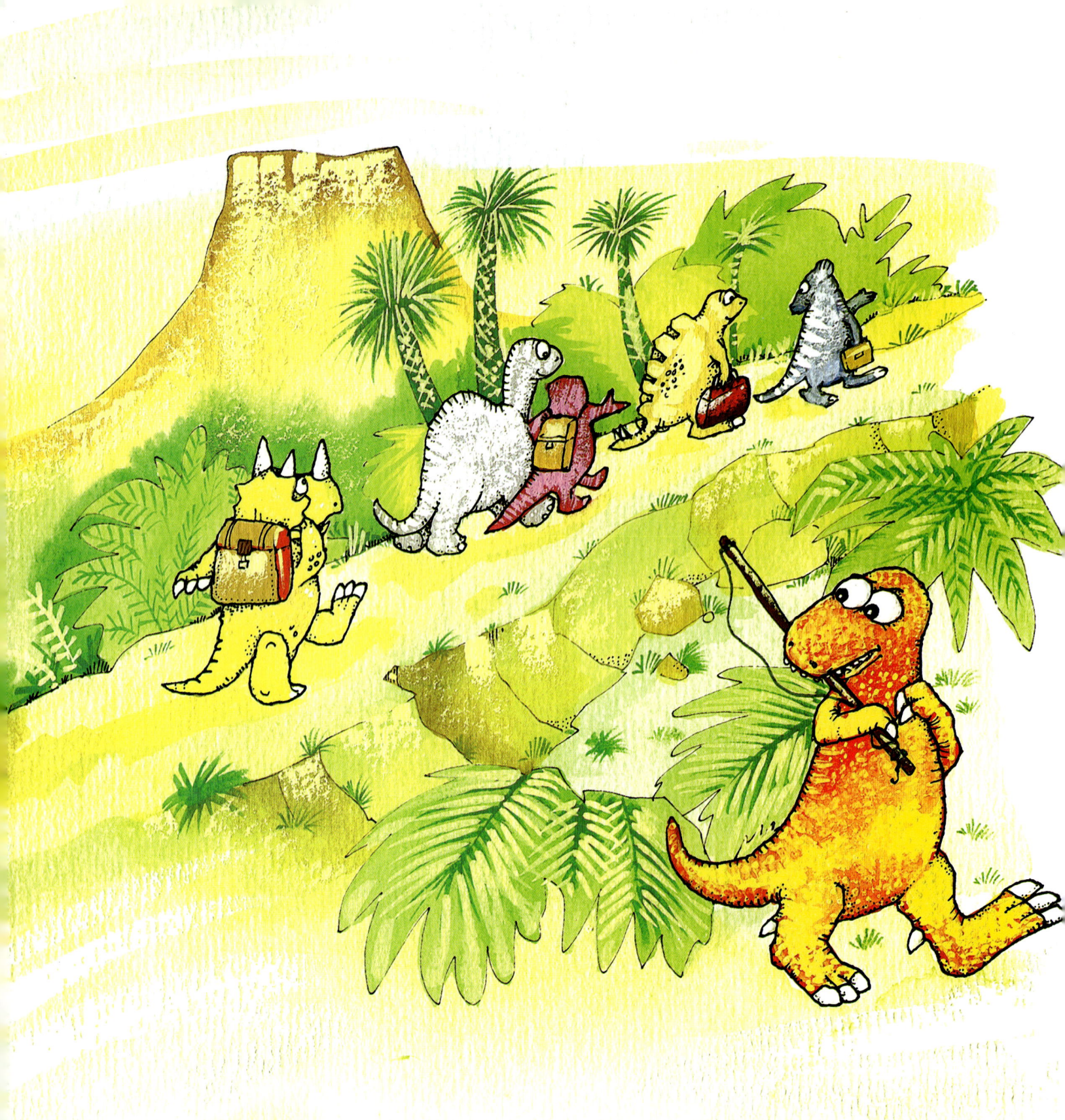

The next day all the young dinosaurs went to school—all except Marvin. Marvin didn't want to go to school. He wanted to go fishing instead!

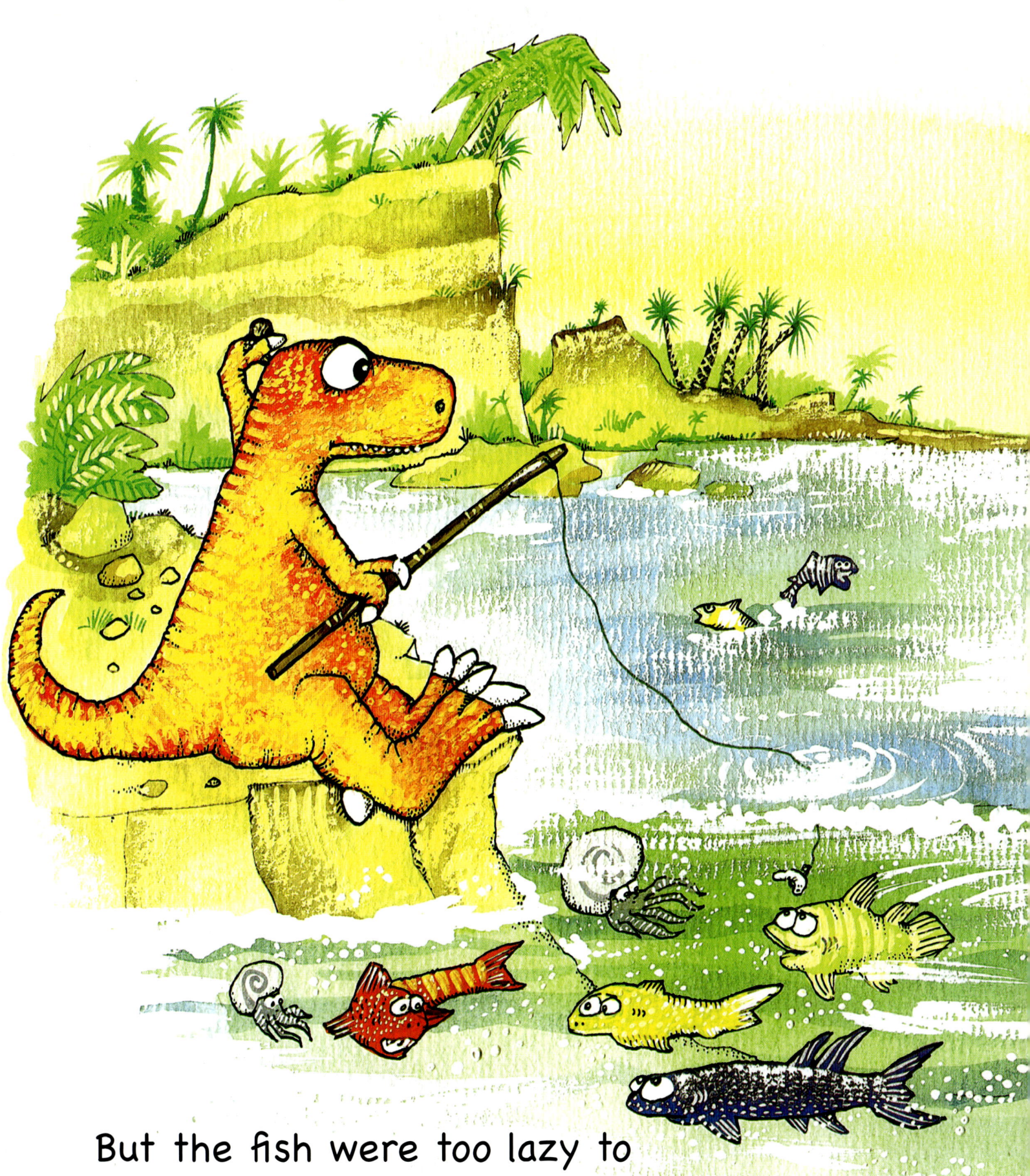

But the fish were too lazy to bite, so Marvin decided to throw pebbles into the water.

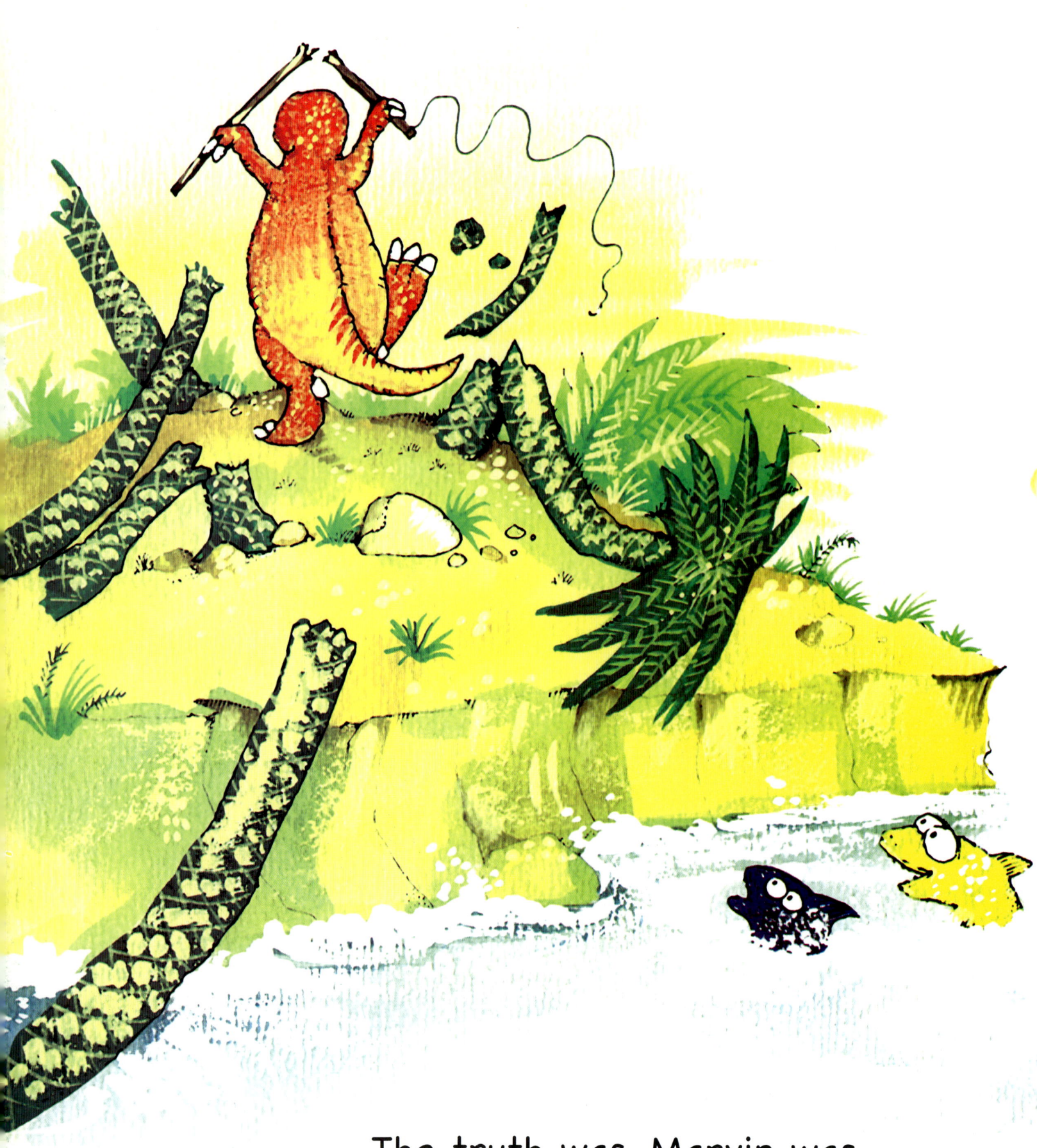

The truth was, Marvin was getting bored very quickly.

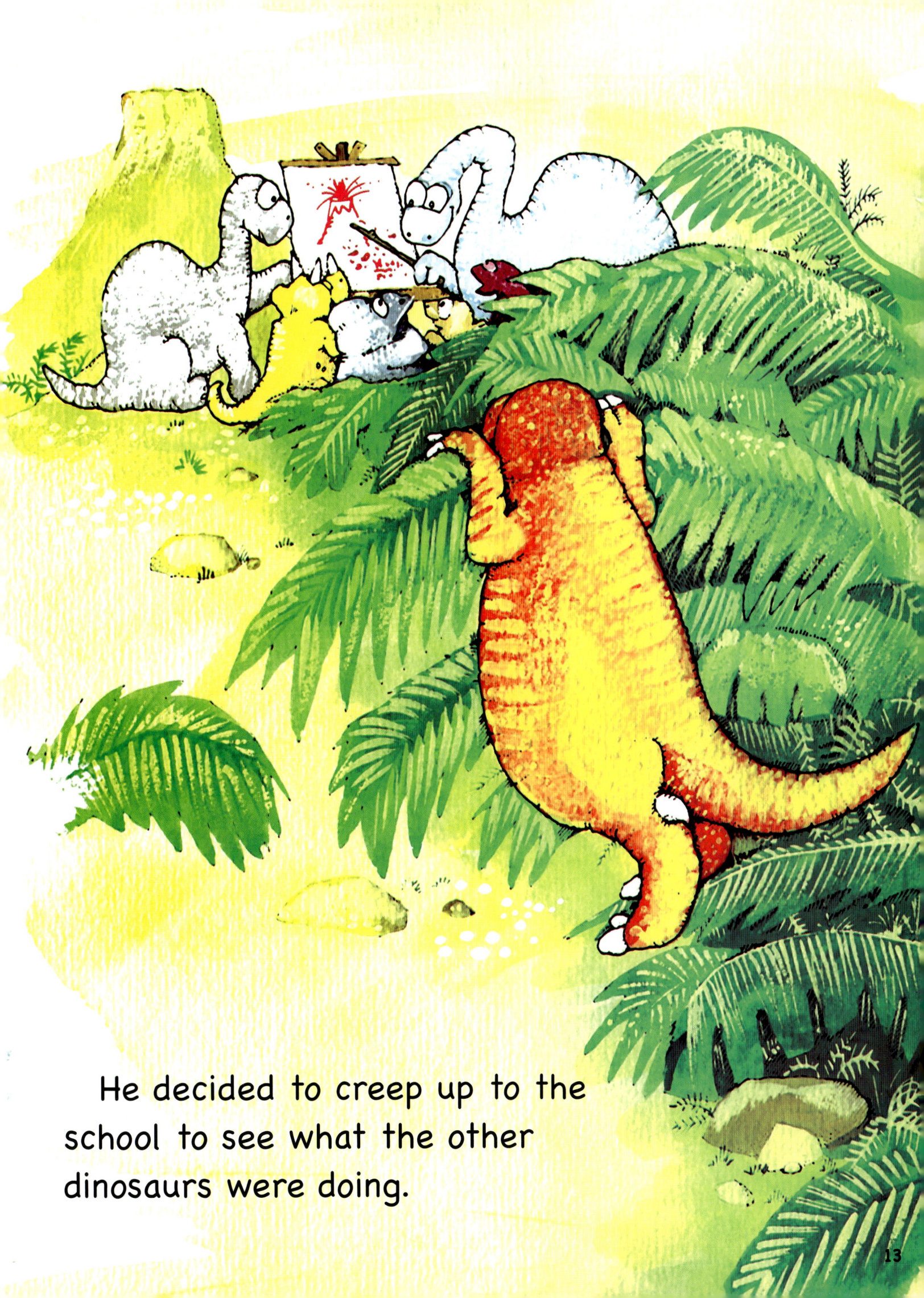

He decided to creep up to the school to see what the other dinosaurs were doing.

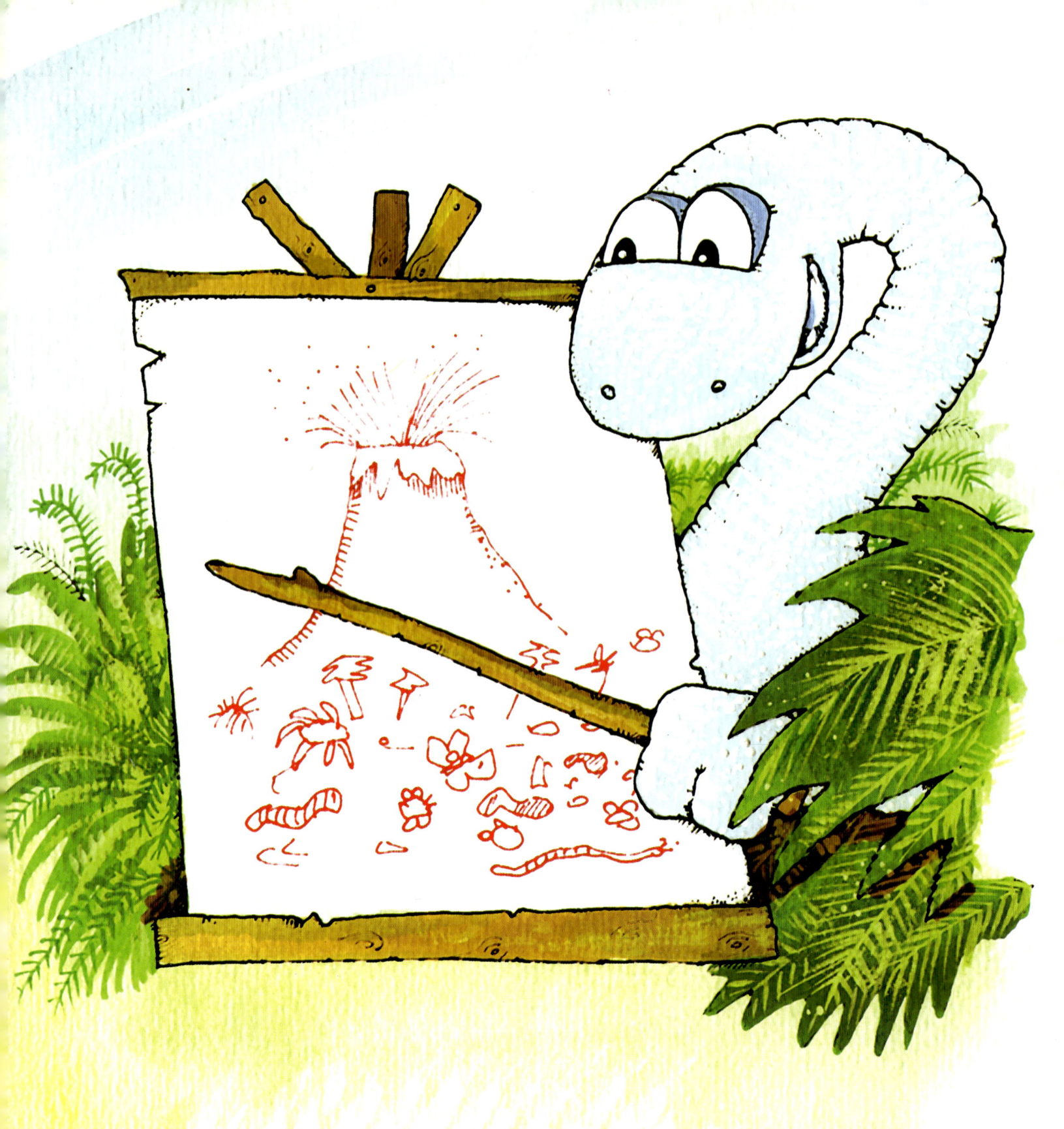

The teacher was about to take the class to the swamp for a lesson on insects and trees.

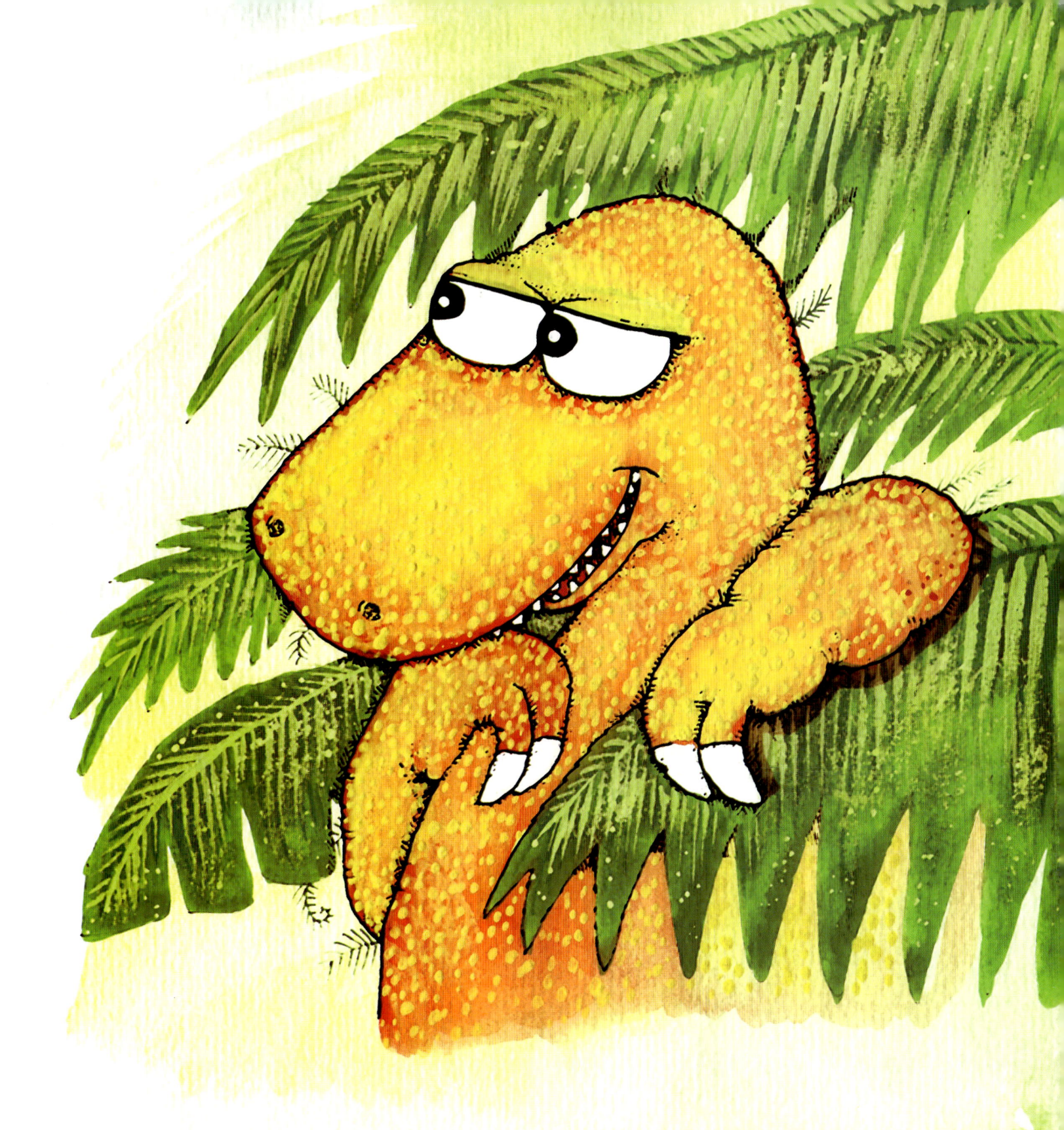

As Marvin listened, a sneaky idea popped into his head. 'I'll play a trick on them!' he thought. 'They'll have a lesson they will never forget!'

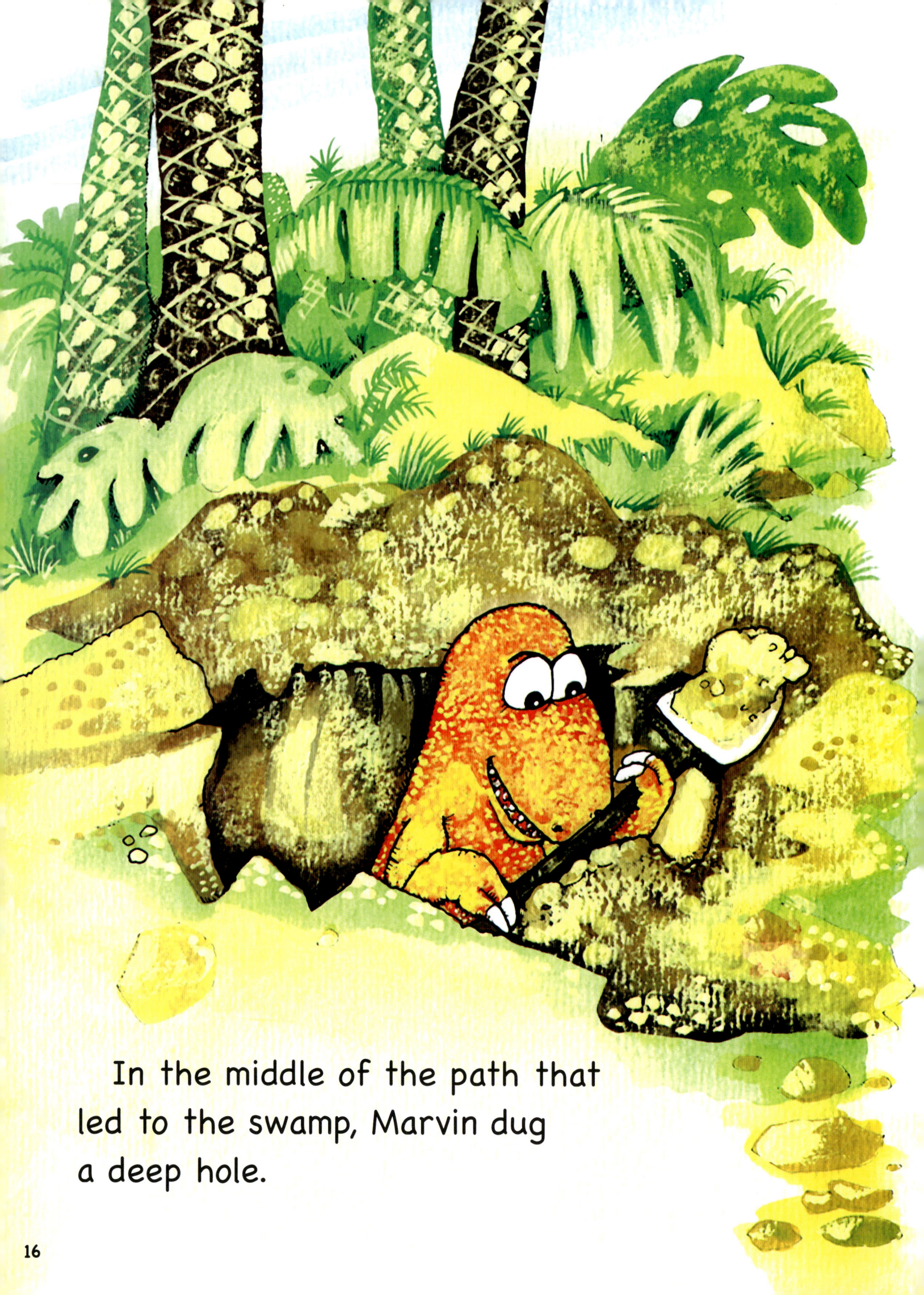

In the middle of the path that led to the swamp, Marvin dug a deep hole.

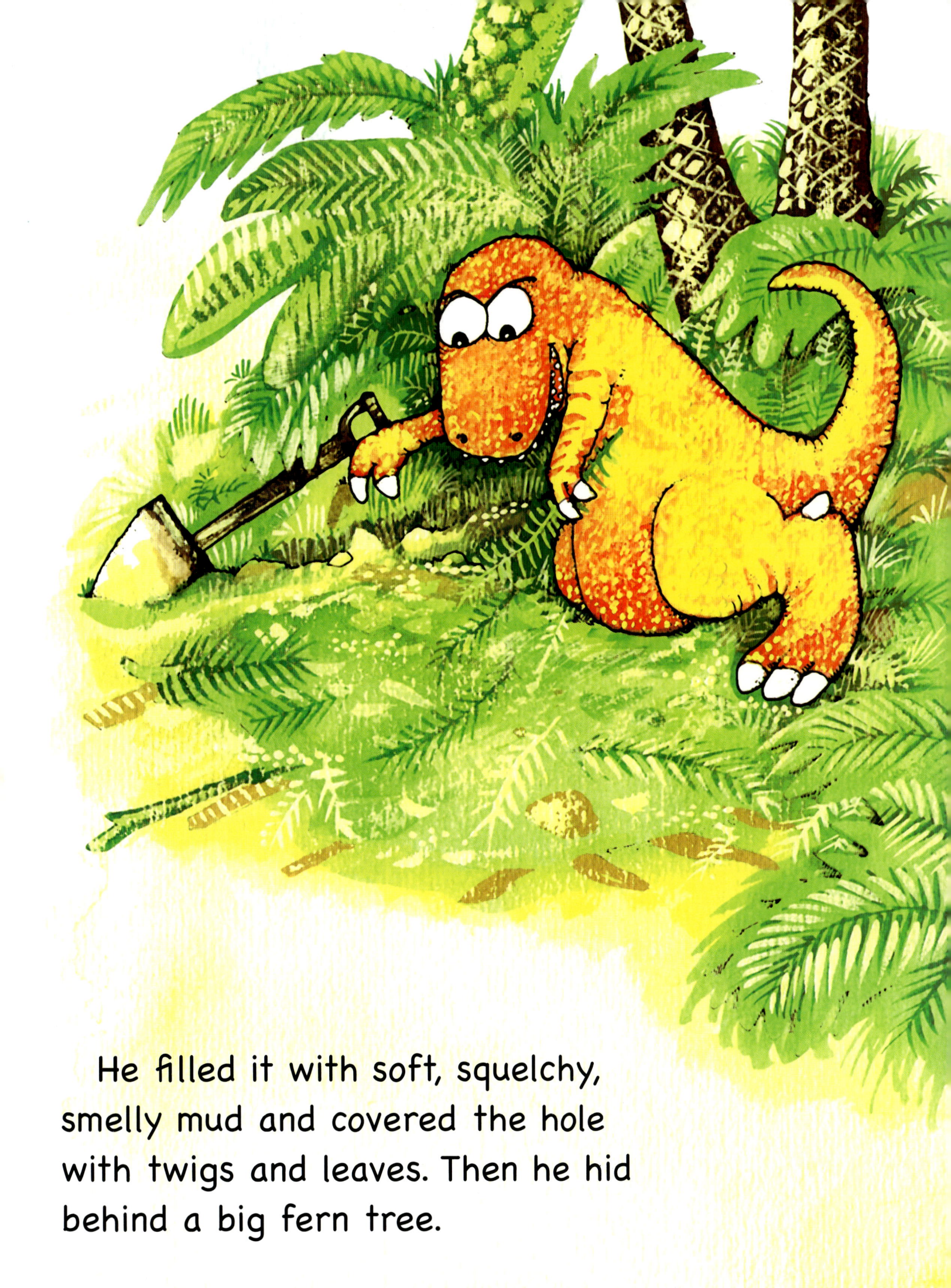

He filled it with soft, squelchy, smelly mud and covered the hole with twigs and leaves. Then he hid behind a big fern tree.

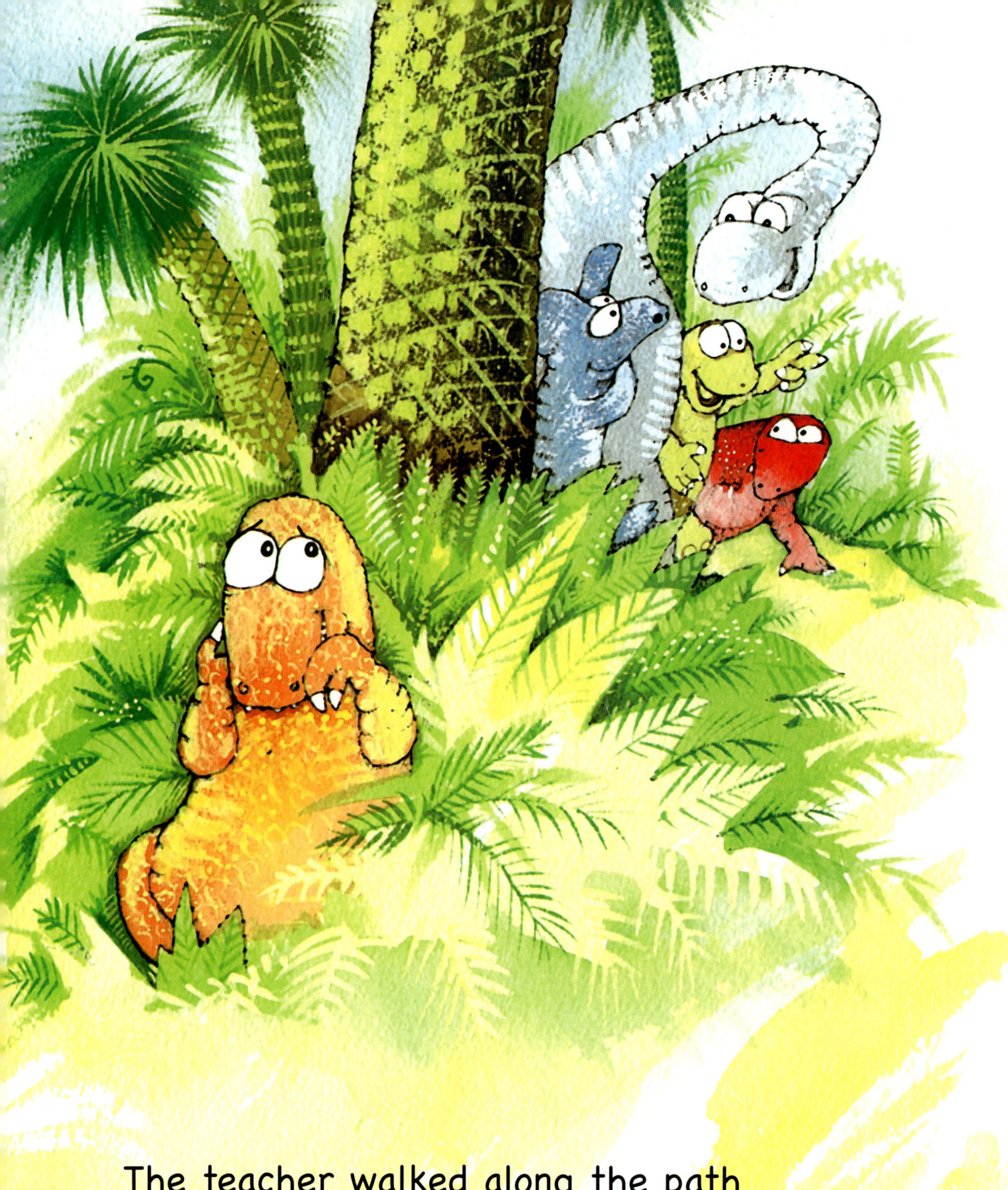

The teacher walked along the path surrounded by the class of young dinosaurs. Marvin could hear them coming closer.

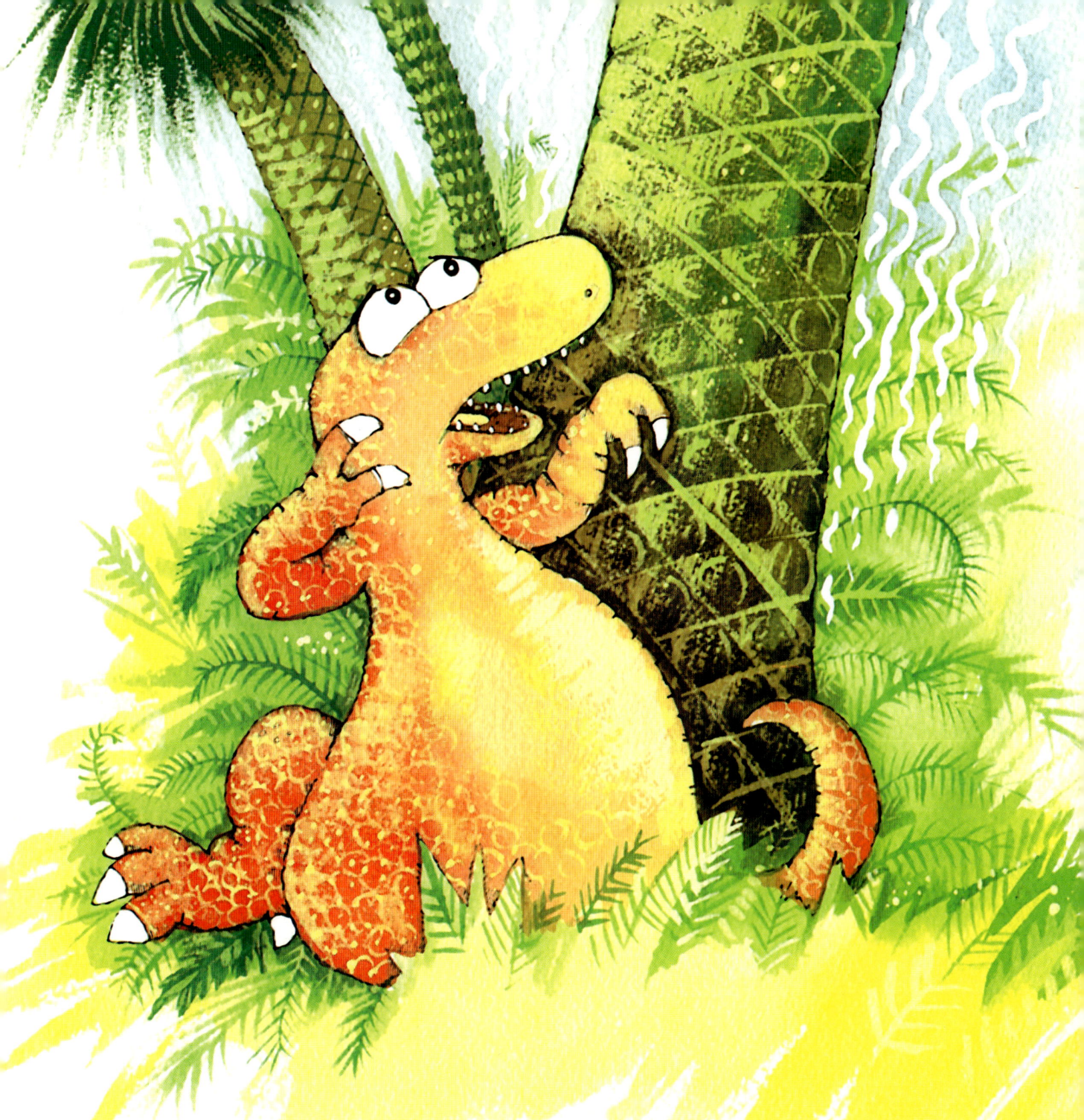

Just before they reached Marvin's mud trap the ground started to tremble and shake. It was an **EARTHQUAKE!**

The big fern tree started to sway dangerously. It was going to fall on the class!

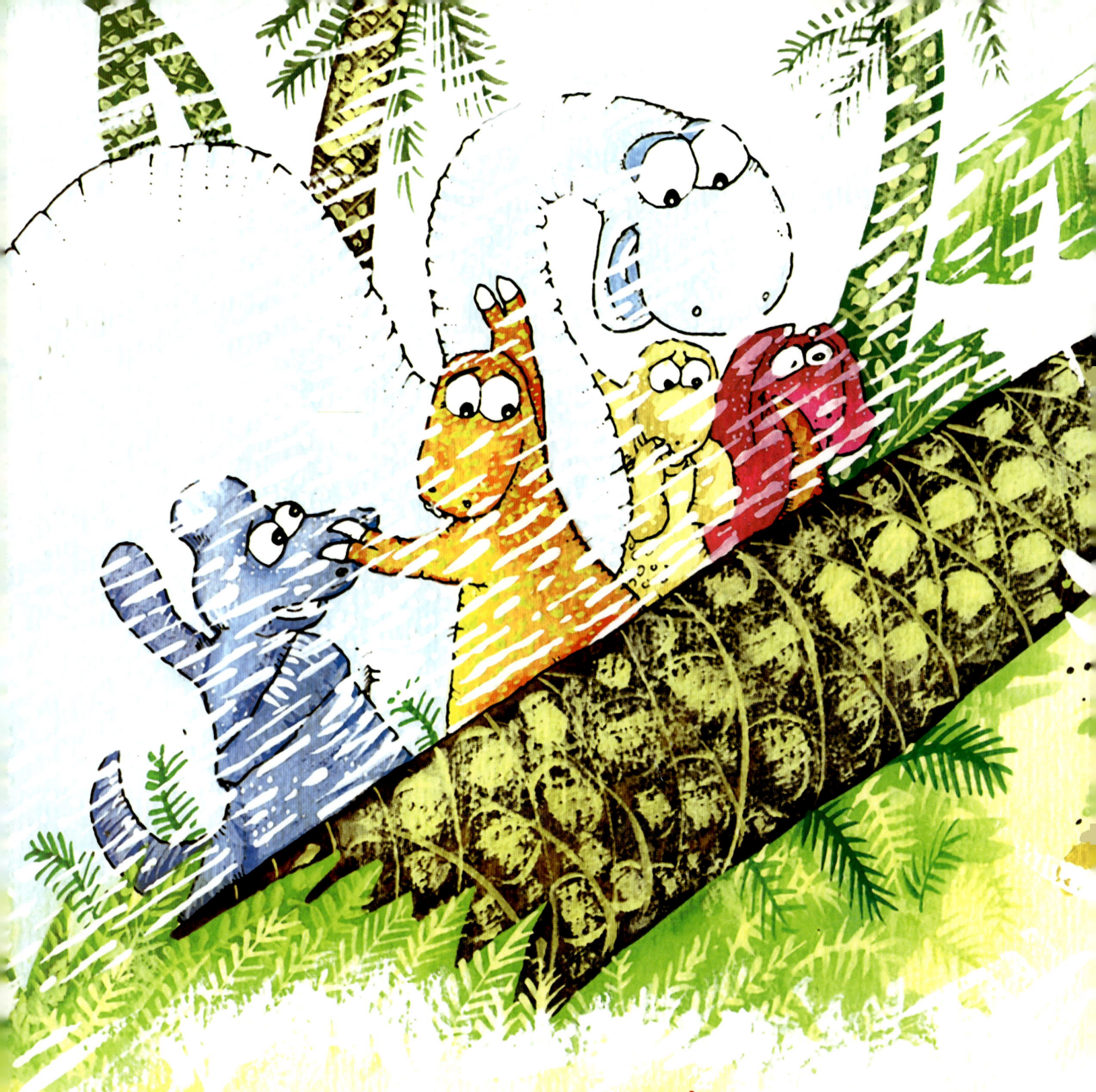

Marvin jumped out shouting, 'GET BACK, GET BACK!'

He pushed the terrified dinosaurs out of the way just seconds before the big tree fern crashed across the path.

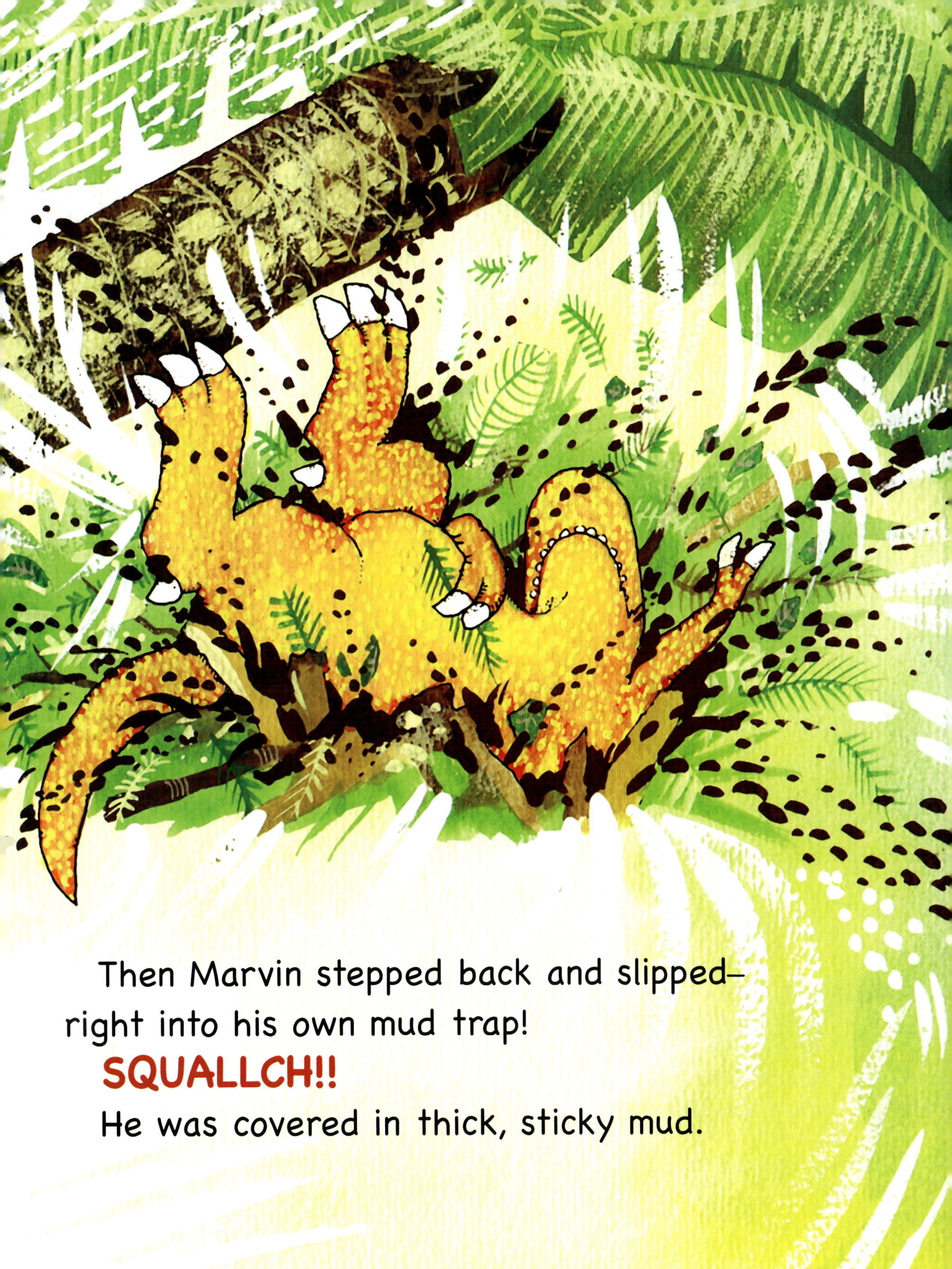

Then Marvin stepped back and slipped—right into his own mud trap!
SQUALLCH!!
He was covered in thick, sticky mud.

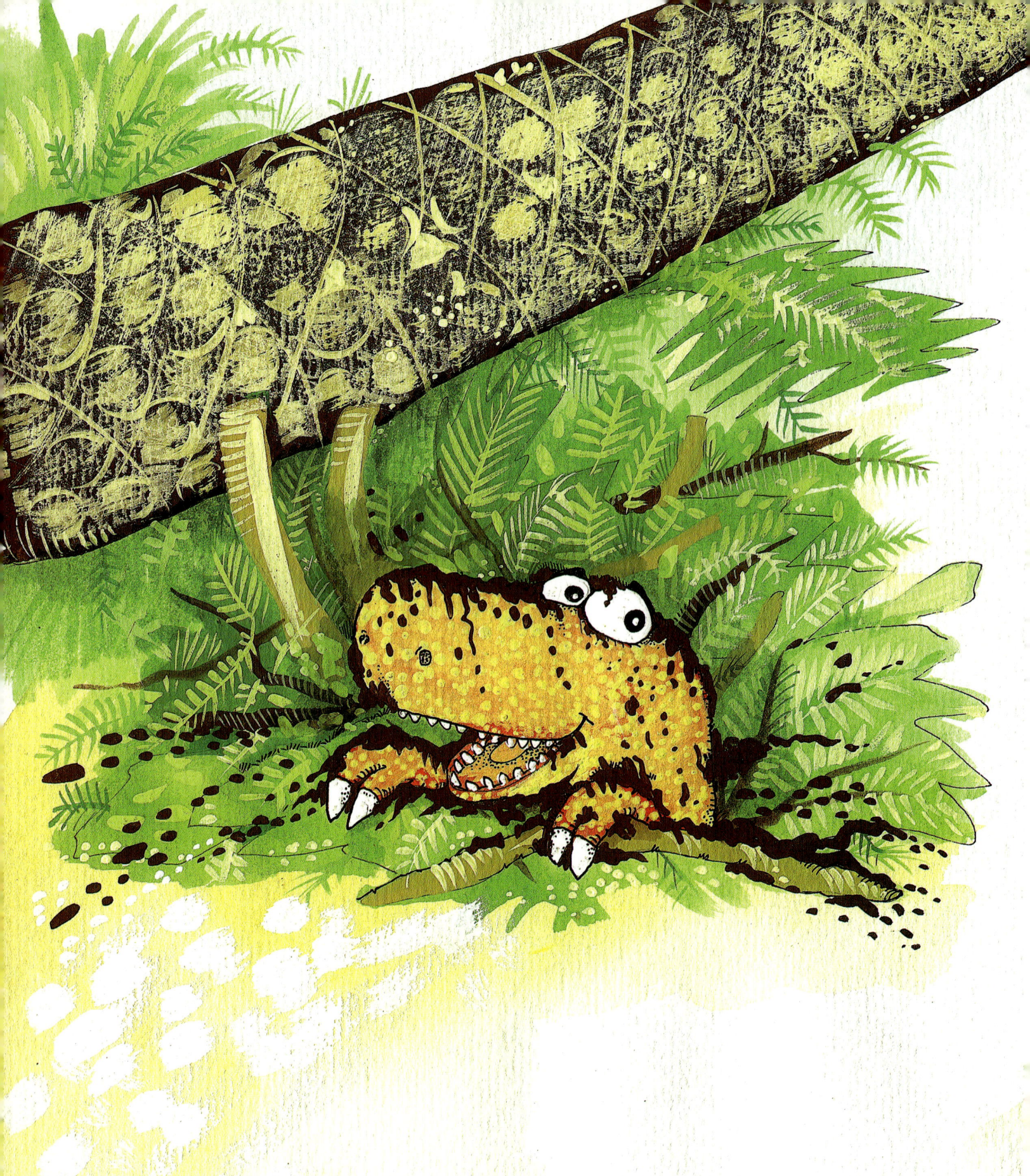

For the first time ever, Marvin didn't lose his temper. Instead, he started to laugh. He was so happy that everyone was safe.

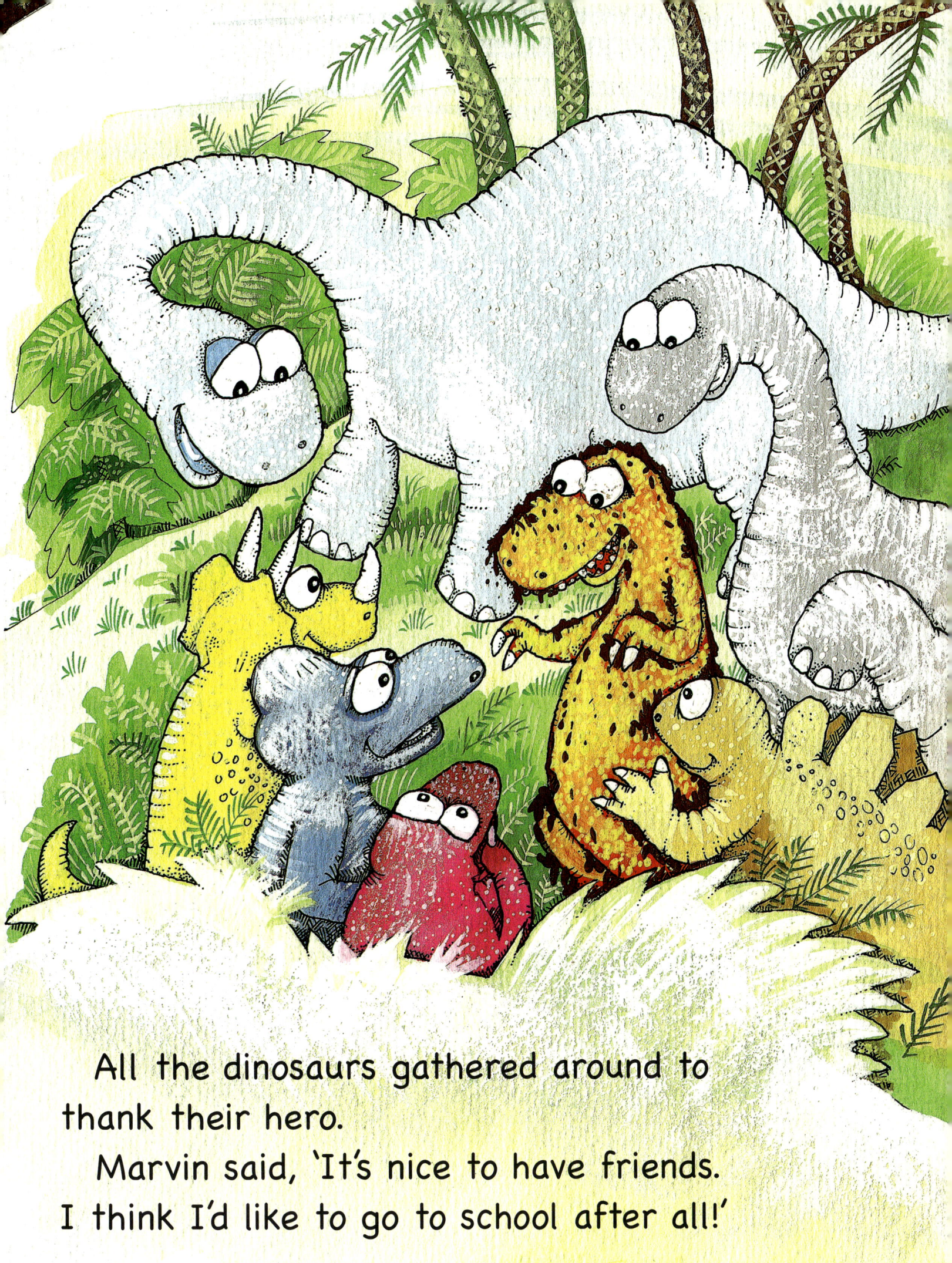

All the dinosaurs gathered around to thank their hero.

Marvin said, 'It's nice to have friends. I think I'd like to go to school after all!'

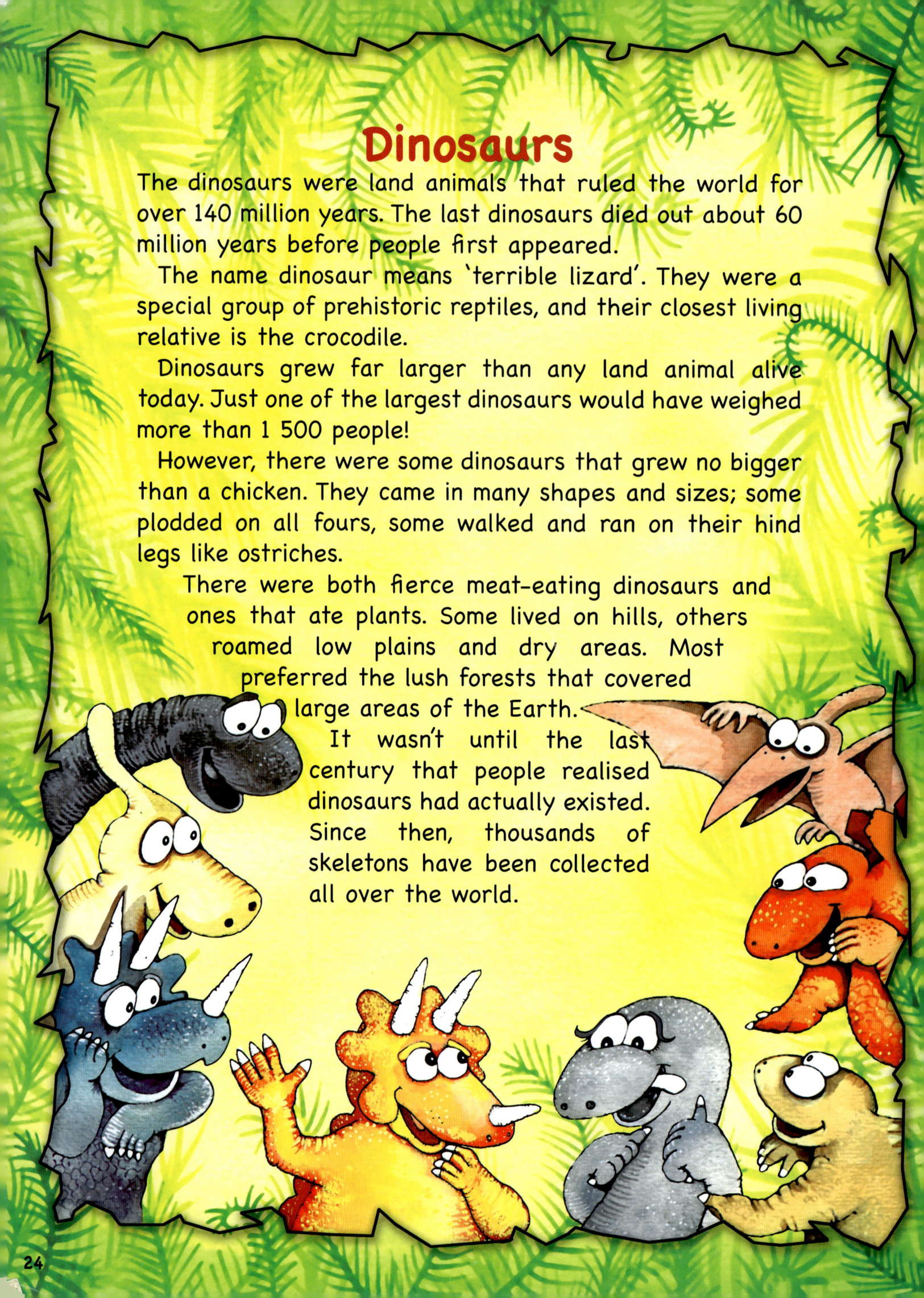

Dinosaurs

The dinosaurs were land animals that ruled the world for over 140 million years. The last dinosaurs died out about 60 million years before people first appeared.

The name dinosaur means 'terrible lizard'. They were a special group of prehistoric reptiles, and their closest living relative is the crocodile.

Dinosaurs grew far larger than any land animal alive today. Just one of the largest dinosaurs would have weighed more than 1 500 people!

However, there were some dinosaurs that grew no bigger than a chicken. They came in many shapes and sizes; some plodded on all fours, some walked and ran on their hind legs like ostriches.

There were both fierce meat-eating dinosaurs and ones that ate plants. Some lived on hills, others roamed low plains and dry areas. Most preferred the lush forests that covered large areas of the Earth.

It wasn't until the last century that people realised dinosaurs had actually existed. Since then, thousands of skeletons have been collected all over the world.